I0436419

IBD DIET

COOKBOOK

100+ Nutrient-Packed recipes for people suffering from Crohn's Diseases, Diverticulitis and Ulcerative Colitis.

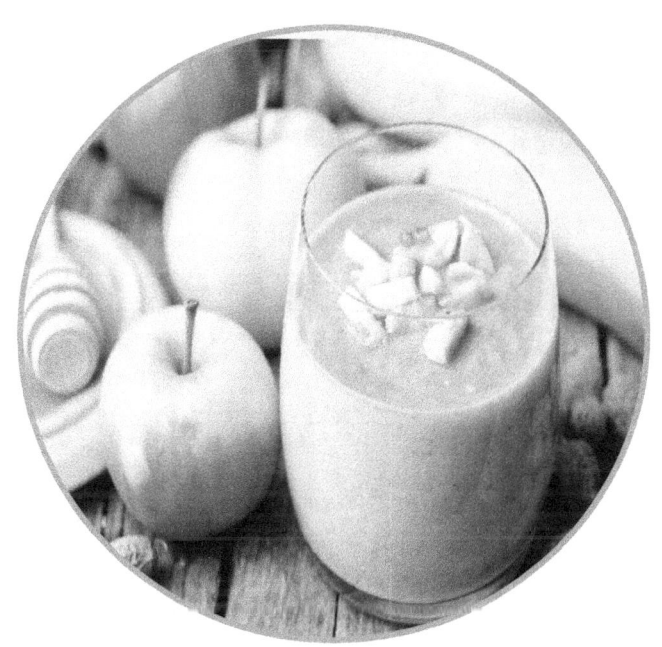

OLIVIA MITCHELL

COPYRIGHT

Table of Contents

INTRODUCTION

Have you ever felt pain in your stomach after eating? Do the fears of being triggered by your IBD prevent you from socializing, as well as dining out at restaurants or trying new foods? Do you find it so exhausting to think of healthy meal preparation and planning?

You're not alone. There are a huge number of people in this world who suffer from IBD like you. However, you don't have to lead a limited life. Imagine a world where you can:

- Enjoy tasty foods, pain-free.
- Ensure that you fuel your body with right nutrients for healing and good health.
- The joy of cooking is back, and you are free to cook and eat with confidence.

That delicious and nutritious reality is yours. That's what this cookbook is your roadmap. We understand the unique challenges individuals with IBD face, and we have made a collection of beginner-friendly recipes that are:

- Essential nutrients and gut-friendly ingredients are rich.
- Prepared easily even with no cooking experience.
- So delicately flavored to titillate your taste buds.
- Free from common IBD triggers.

This book will not only provide you with recipes but also help you relate how nutrients contribute to IBD. You'll learn about:

- Specific nutrients that can help manage inflammation and promote healing.
- Foods to avoid and healthy substitutes to embrace.
- Essential tips for planning and preparing meals that nourish your body and soul.
- Strategies for managing stress and optimizing your overall well-being.

My journey with IBD began when I was diagnosed in my early twenties. Frustrated by the lack of accessible and reliable information, I embarked on a mission to learn everything I could about the disease and its dietary needs. Through years of research, experimentation, and collaboration with healthcare professionals, I have developed a personalized approach to managing my IBD through delicious and nutritious food.

This is my passion project, the fruit of many years of studying and learning in order to help you achieve health and happiness for yourself. Now turn the next page and start your culinary journey. As a team, let us make a difference and the way you eat, feel, and live with IBD.

CHAPTER 1

What You Should Know About Ibd

In order to effectively plan and make the right decisions along the ride, it is important to have an understanding of the terrain on which we will travel. This chapter will introduce you to Inflammatory Bowel Disease (IBD) and answer some fundamental questions:

- What exactly is IBD?
- What are the different types of IBD?
- What are the causes and symptoms of IBD?
- How is IBD diagnosed and treated?

What is IBD?

Inflammatory bowel disease is a group of chronic intestinal inflammatory diseases which leads to destruction of tissues in gut wall. Such inflammation causes several unpleasant and incapacitating symptoms which will affect your everyday life.

How Does Diet Affect IBD?

Food is not only sustenance for the body. It is a potent instrument that may either aggravate or control the impacts of different diseases such as IBD. To be therefore precise; what role does diet play in IBD?

7

1. Gut-Brain Connection:

- Your gut and your brain talk all the time.
- The type of food you eat signals your cell, which in turn affects immune responses and digestion.
- Some dietary constituents allow healthy gut bacteria to grow.
- Other food types support unwholesome bacteria in such a way that they cause an inflammatory response that eventually leads to tissue destruction.

2. Food as Information:

- Your gut views food as informational, and it affects gene expression and determines general wellbeing.
- These include essential nutrients like antioxidants, vitamins, and healthy fats.
- Inflammation is easily aggravated by such ingredients found in processed food.

3. Targeted Nutrition for IBD:

- Feeding good gut bacteria is accomplished by increasing fiber intake.
- For instance, Omega-3 fatty acids, fruits, and vegetables are anti-inflammatory foods.

- Eliminating processed foods decreases the consumption of bad nutrients.2

- Some have experienced significant improvement of their symptoms through a low-FODMAP diet.

Knowing which foods aggravate or worsen your IBD allows you to select dietary options that suit your case better.

The subsequent chapter shall discuss certain nutrients required by a patient suffering from IBD, as well as the identification of trigger foods.

Picture yourself leading a life with no food wars; rather, a friend in need in your war against health problems. An IBD food plan is a tailored route through difficult waters in your gut that has the power. So, buckle up, because we're about to explore the benefits that await you on this delicious journey:

1. Symptom Relief: From Roar to Purr

Sick of explosive reactions upon digesting one's food in one's system as though you're a rumbling volcano after every meal? The fire extinguishers will work like IBD diet and calm down the inflammatory fuel for all those symptoms you don't feel like! The gut's happy feeling less abdominal pain, fewer urgent trips to the bathroom, and think to healthy lifestyle.

2. Energy Boost: From Lag to Leap

Ever felt like a withered flower on a sunny day? Energy and fatigue are common complaints of IBD patients. However, eating healthy nutrients that promote good bacteria for your insides could be your true sunshine that fills up your tank and allows you to stride into that summer of yours.

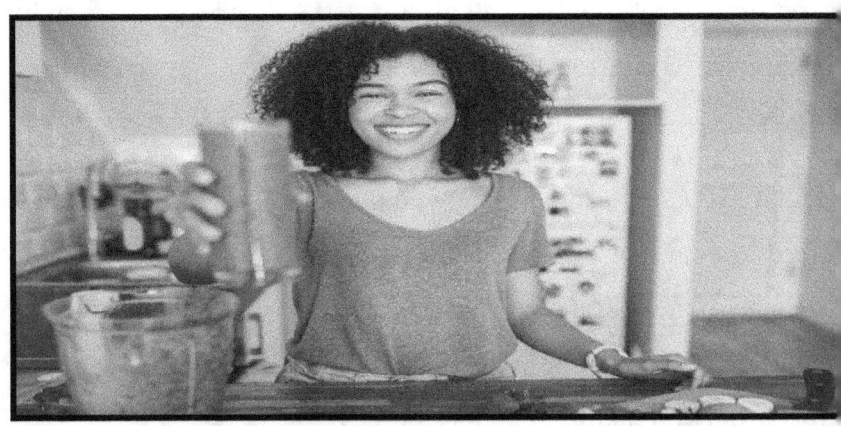

3. Improved Mood: sunshine smile from a grumpy cloud.

It is not a myth that the gut talks to the brain. You know, what you eat may even affect one's mood." A diet of IBD high in mood boosting nutrients can clear out the haze of fatigue and restlessness allowing your sunshine to come out.

4. Reduced Risk of Complications:

Your IBD should be viewed as a shield against possible complications. Reduction of the risks that come with infection or surgery by reducing inflammations. Similar to creating an armadillo for your intestine but with delectable bites along the way.

5. Empowerment and Control:

IBD is a condition that can leave you feeling like you have no control over your own body. However, an IBD diet puts you back at the wheel. Informing yourself on what you eat equips you with power over your own health that lets you take charge.

6. Discovering Delicious New Adventures:

Do not allow IBD to limit what you eat. The IBD diet is about discovery not deprivation. That's the discovery of the new world of healthy, tasty foods for your tummy and your body. Spice up your life with spicy stir-fries, avocado dips and fiber-rich smoothies.

Just note that the benefits of IBD diet depend on you, just like personality is unique for everyone. The changes will happen gradually for some people while other people may experience significant remission of their symptoms. But one thing's for sure: each of your munch will be a mile forward in health and happiness.

Hence, are you all prepared for this mouth-watering journey? The chapter to follow will delve into the IBD nutrition, focusing especially on the nutrients to live on for the recovery and the ones to skip out on.

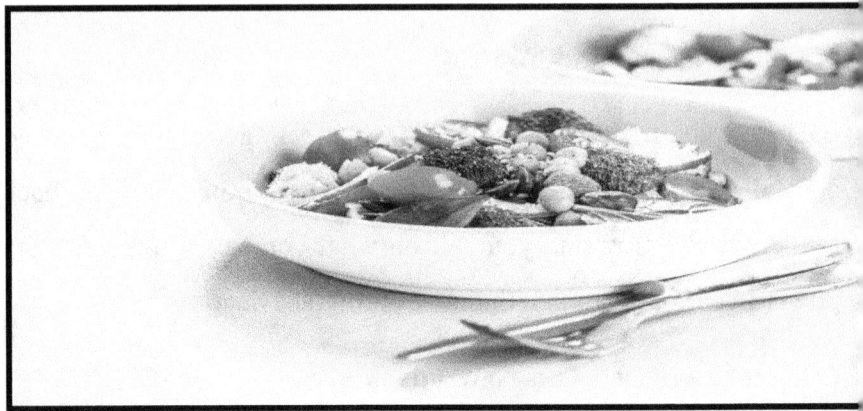

CHAPTER 2

Foods To Avoid

Picture your gut as a quiet garden full of beautiful flowers and animals. However, amidst all the stunning surroundings come some undesirable guests – foods that stir up a lot of trouble in the form of inflammation and discomfort for those with IBD. Thus, get you a comfortable map and let's venture into "Food Minefields", pointing out mine and learning the turf.

1. The Spicy Sentries:

Although a hot kick may excite your tongue, certain IBD warriors consider spice the same as an armed guard blocking access to their intestines. Even chilis, pepper, and some other spices such as garlic and paprika can make things worse by irritating the gut lining leading to inflammation and exacerbating the symptoms. But fear not, spice lovers! Try the softer ways such as ginger, turmeric and other herbs that give great flavors without being extreme.

2. The Fatty Foes:

Consider greasy and fried foods like the heavy artillery in the food minefield. It may be difficult for you to metabolize them, stress up your stomach, and cause inflammation of cells. Although, some delights like deep-fried foods, meat and fatty sauces should be restricted. Healthy fats (e.g., avocado/olive oil), lean protein dishes (grilled or baked) can be chosen as great alternatives for them.

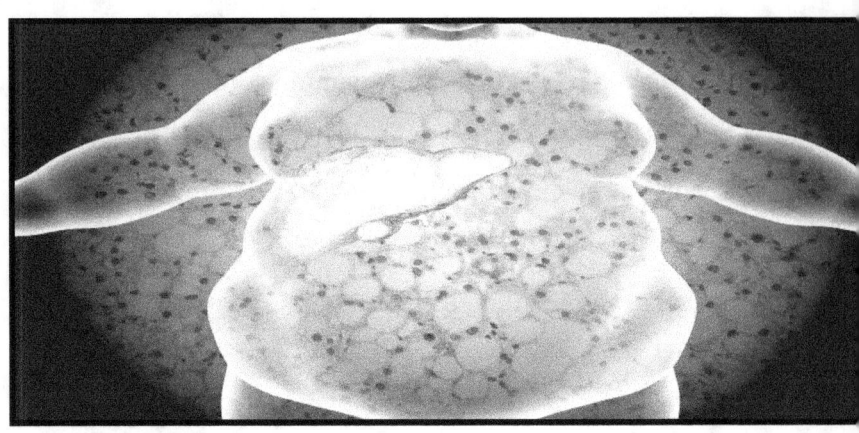

3. The FODMAP Frenzy:

As some IBD warriors discover, their bellies become riddled with gas when they eat particular small gnomes called FODMAPS which are some types of fermentable carbohydrates. These hidden sugars include those contained in pears, apples and many similar products and even some dairy foods. However, not all FODMAPs are problematic. Try and identify your personal tolerable amounts and look for low FODMAP substitutes as a strategy to maintain your happier gut.

4. The Lactose Lurkers:

Lactose is another hidden enemy for others. In many instances, lactose intolerant patients or those having IBD may become distressed due to this as their abdomens are most vulnerable and liable areas of the digestive system.y Ensure that there are no lactose lurkers by exploring lactose-free milk options, plant-based milks like almond or soy, as well as mouthwatering lactose-free yogurts and cheese alternatives.

5. The Fiber Faux Pas:

Fiber is hailed as a gut hero and while that may be true for many people, it could prove harmful for individuals suffering from IBD. Some high-fiber foods such as uncooked/undigested vegetables, nuts, seeds, etc., could also trigger or aggravate IBS symptoms. However, always keep in mind that you need fiber too! To enjoy the benefits of fiber without feeling uncomfortable, go for well-cooked or finely chopped vegetables; ground nuts and seeds; and whole grains sparingly.

It is important to remember that it is the Food Minefield of IBD of each individual. Something that an individual may tolerate might affect someone else adversely. Listen to your body, do experiments and discover the method that suits you in the best way possible. This cookbook will be your guide and company providing wholesome gut friendly recipes and navigation skills through the territory.

Common food triggers for IBD symptoms

Does it ever feel as though you were a detective following after every meal in an attempt to decipher your IBD symptom's mystery? You're not alone! Our kitchen cupboards are often swarming with numerous potential culprits who could set off gastrointestinal problems. Oh, but you need not worry, fellow food detectives! This chapter is your magnifying glass, helping you identify the common culprits and build a personalized "No-Go List" for your gut:

1. The Spicy Suspects:

In this case, chilis, peppers, and even garlic can be as fiery as villains that set your digestive track ablaze. Their capsaicin content could cause stomach ache due to erosion of the gut lining. It may sound difficult to wave good bye to these hot bomb flavors but there are better spices such as turmeric, ginger, and herbs that could bring in a sweet spicy touch to your meal.

2. The Fatty Foes:

Greasy goons are roaming around in the kitchen looking for greasy foods such as deep-fried delights, fatty meat, and creamy sauces because they overload your stomach causing inflammation to worsen. Go for healthier options like grilled chicken or fish, baked foods, and good fats such as avocados' and olive oil to make your tummies happy while satisfying your buds.

3. The FODMAP Phantoms:

Sneaky sugars are found in such fruits as apples and cherries, vegetables like onions and garlic, and even dairy products. Don't fret! Find out how much FODMAP you can tolerate and search for FODMAP free options which include berries, leafy green vegetables, gluten-free grain substitutes, etc.

4. The Lactose Lurkers:

Some people with IBD view lactose, a substance found in milk as a secret culprit that instigates stomach upsets. However, this "dairy detective" should not scare you off. Be open to lactose-free milks such as almond or soy and yummy lactose-free yoghurts and cheese which will leave your gut in smiles.

5. The Fructose Faux Pas:

However, fructose (natural sugar) could also turn out to be a cunning hero. Fruits as a rule go easy on the stomach, but large quantities of fructose for some people trigger discomfort because of irritable bowel disease (IBD). Find out your own tolerance point, but also look at other options such as fruit substitutes like bananas or melons that have less fructose content.

Note that recognizing your own triggers requires a process and not an event per se. And this chapter is merely an introduction. Keep food diary, listen to your body, and work your health care team in order to make your refined "No-go list". More you will understand your Gut's language, more empowered you will have in navigating culinary territory with confidence knowing good meals won't harm.

CHAPTER 3

Foods To Eat

Say bye-bye to boring food choices and dietary restrictions! In the "Food Oasis", your body begins to feed on a delightful gastronomical journey. This combines deliciousness and a gut friendly magic allowing you to eat well en route to your IBD mission. Let's explore this haven of nutrient-rich heroes, ready to become the allies your body craves.

Nutrient-Rich Foods For People With IBD

However, "Food Oasis" goes further than making explosion of flavors. Your organism is ready to survive! Think of these nutrient-rich heroes as tiny superheroes, each with a specific power to fuel your IBD journey:

1. Vitamin A: The Gut Lining Guardian:

Think of Vitamin A like a manual worker repairing and reinforcing the wall or barriers in your intestine. Their favorite building blocks include sweet potatoes as well as carrots and leafy green like kales. When it comes to digestion, a good gut lining should lead to lesser problems such as inflammations. And for sure, your stomach should be happy!

2. Vitamin C: The Immune System Booster:

See Vitamin C as a superhero's cape protecting you from infections, fortifying your immune system. Oranges and grapefruit constitute their training ground as well as bell pepper and even broccoli. The immune system acts as part of the body's defense mechanism towards undesired agents that may make one sick.

3. Vitamin D: The Inflammation Fighter:

Imagine that vitamin D is like a relaxing hand which calms down inflammation within all the regions of your body. Their sunny castles are made up of mushrooms and fortified milk. Vitamin D reduces inflammation, decreases joint pain, and improves general health.

4. Omega-3 Fatty Acids: The Anti-Inflammatory Champions:

Think of omega-3 fatty acids as modern knights wearing armor and combating inflammation wherever it appears. Their mighty steeds are fatty fish like salmon or tuna and plant based as chia seeds and walnuts. They decrease gut inflammation, boost your mood and protect your heart by omega-3s.

5. Zinc: The Gut Healing Warrior:

Think of zinc like an experienced nurse who tapes up your ripped and perforated insides. Their operating rooms could be oysters and lean meats. A healthy digestive system can only be achieved through the involvement of zinc which helps in repair of tissues and healing of wounds.

6. Magnesium: The Relaxation Master:

Magnetic is an analgesic balm which takes away muscles pains and helps you fall asleep. They find their respite in leafy greens and nuts. Magnesium helps to ease the gut muscles and thus relieving pain while ensuring the smooth movement of food through the digestive system.

7. Iron: The Energy Energizer:

Think of Iron like a battery for your body. When they eat lentils of beans, it serves as an iron-fuel station. It fights against fatigue in the body thus makes sure that one's energy level is kept at a high state and that the body works as it should.

8. Probiotics: The Gut Flora Guardians:

Visualize probiotics as little gnomes working on your gut garden and cultivating beneficial microbes to flourish. Their lively villages provide fermented delicacies such as yogurt, kimchi, and sauerkraut. It facilitates in preservation of a balance between the beneficial and detrimental intestinal microflora required for proper nutrition, resistance against infections and improved psychological condition.

Never forget that they are more than that. Experience the "Food oasis"; play with flavors and tastes while treating your physical body to a delectable sensation in every bite. Your pathway to a healthy gut, seasoned with flavors powered through enriched dietary sources.

The following chapter will take us on a journey to lunch-time, where practicality and gut friendly treats collide. Brace for some inventive, delectably healthy ways to keep you satisfied till dusk.

CHAPTER 4

Breakfast Recipes

A tummy filling breakfast rich in nutrients is good for people with IBD as it provides them with energy. Breakfast goes beyond just eating, but rather provides the required energy needed by the body to deal with another day in the office. This chapter has ten healthy breakfast recipes for use by any individual suffering with IBD as part of a strategy to boost their general health. [...] The IBD warriors should have different tastes of foods as they break the fast. From gentle and easily digestive foods, which are also rich in energy, to nutritious ones that provide power for them.

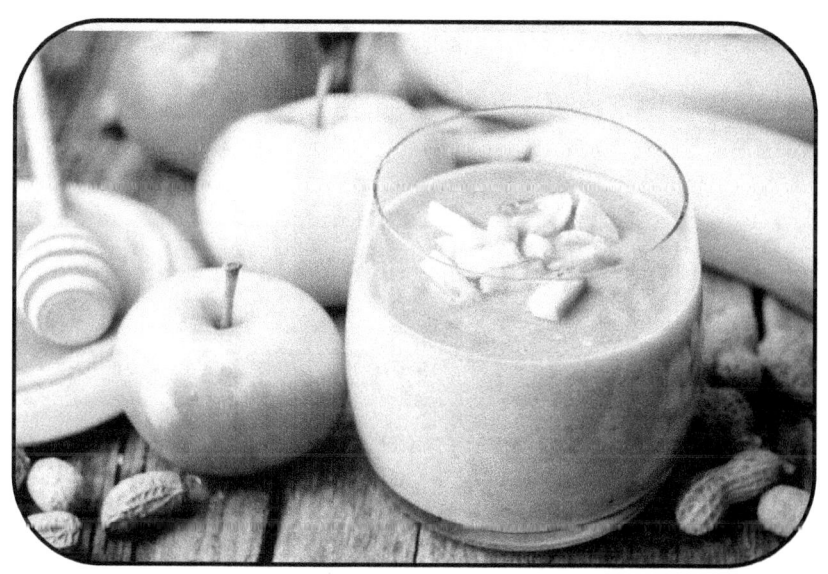

1. Creamy Sunrise Smoothie

Ingredients:

- 1 cup frozen mango chunks
- 1/2 teaspoon turmeric powder
- 1/2 inch fresh ginger, grated
- 1 cup kefir (or unsweetened almond milk)
- 1 handful fresh spinach

Instructions:

- Combine all ingredients in a blender and blend until smooth and creamy.
- Enjoy immediately for a refreshing and gut-friendly start to your day.

2. Protein-Packed Power Pancakes

Ingredients:

- 1/2 cup rolled oats
- 2 tablespoons chia seeds
- 1 scoop protein powder (optional)
- 1/2 cup unsweetened almond milk
- 1/4 teaspoon baking powder

- Pinch of salt
- Berries and honey for topping (optional)

Instructions:

- In a medium bowl, whisk together oats, chia seeds, protein powder (if using), baking powder, and salt.
- Add almond milk and stir until a thick batter forms. Let sit for 5 minutes to thicken further.
- Heat a lightly greased skillet over medium heat. Pour batter into small rounds, cooking for 2-3 minutes per side until golden brown and fluffy.
- Top with berries and honey (if using) and enjoy a satisfying protein-rich breakfast.

3. Savory Scrambled Eggs with Spinach and Avocado

Ingredients:

- 2 eggs
- 1/4 teaspoon turmeric powder
- Pinch of garlic powder
- 1 handful fresh spinach
- 1/4 avocado, sliced
- Olive oil for cooking

Instructions:

- In a small bowl, whisk together eggs, turmeric, and garlic powder.
- Heat a drizzle of olive oil in a skillet over medium heat. Add spinach and cook until wilted.
- Pour in the egg mixture and scramble until just set.
- Top with sliced avocado and enjoy a protein-packed and gut-friendly breakfast.

4. Baked Sweet Potato Hash with Poached Egg:

Ingredients:

- 1 medium sweet potato, diced
- 1 bell pepper, diced (any color)
- 1/2 red onion, diced
- 1 tablespoon olive oil
- 1/4 teaspoon smoked paprika
- Salt and pepper to taste
- 1 egg
- Vinegar or lemon juice

Instructions:

- Preheat oven to 400°F (200°C). Toss sweet potato, bell pepper, and onion with olive oil, paprika, salt, and pepper.
- Spread on a baking sheet and bake for 20-25 minutes, or until tender.
- While the hash bakes, bring a pot of water to a simmer. Add vinegar or lemon juice.
- Crack an egg into a small bowl. Swirl the water to create a vortex and carefully drop the egg into the center. Cook for 3-4 minutes, or until the whites are set and the yolk is still runny.
- Spoon the baked hash onto a plate and top with the poached egg. Enjoy a vibrant and gut-friendly breakfast bowl.

5. Overnight Chia Seed Pudding with Berries and Nuts

Ingredients:

- 1/4 cup chia seeds
- 1 cup unsweetened almond milk
- 1/2 teaspoon vanilla extract
- Honey or maple syrup to taste (optional)
- 1/2 cup fresh berries
- 1/4 cup chopped nuts

Instructions:

- In a jar or container, whisk together chia seeds, almond milk, vanilla extract, and honey or maple syrup (if using). Cover and refrigerate overnight.
- In the morning, stir in fresh berries and chopped nuts. Enjoy a fiber-rich and gut-friendly breakfast on the go.

6. Banana-Oatmeal Smoothie with Almond Butter:

Ingredients:

- 1 frozen banana
- 1/2 cup rolled oats
- 1 tablespoon almond butter
- 1 cup unsweetened almond milk
- Pinch of cinnamon

Instructions:

- Combine all ingredients in a blender and blend until smooth and creamy.
- Enjoy this gut-friendly smoothie for a quick and energizing breakfast.

7. Green Smoothie with Spinach, Kale, and Banana

Ingredients:

- 1 handful fresh spinach
- 1 handful fresh kale
- 1 frozen banana
- 1 cup unsweetened almond milk
- 1 scoop protein powder (optional)
- 1/2 teaspoon vanilla extract
- Pinch of ginger (optional)

Instructions:

- Combine all ingredients in a blender and blend until smooth and creamy.
- Enjoy this vitamin-packed and gut-friendly smoothie for a refreshing and energizing start to your day.

8. Scrambled Tofu with Turmeric and Bell Peppers

Ingredients:

- 1/2 block firm tofu, drained and crumbled
- 1/4 teaspoon turmeric powder
- Pinch of garlic powder
- 1/2 cup bell peppers (any color), diced
- 1/4 cup chopped onion
- Olive oil for cooking
- Fresh parsley for garnish (optional)

Instructions:

- In a medium bowl, toss crumbled tofu with turmeric and garlic powder.
- Heat a drizzle of olive oil in a skillet over medium heat. Add onions and cook until softened.
- Add bell peppers and cook until slightly tender.
- Add tofu and cook, stirring occasionally, until heated through and slightly browned.
- Garnish with fresh parsley (if using) and enjoy a plant-based and gut-friendly breakfast scramble.

9. Baked Apples with Cinnamon and Walnuts:

Ingredients:

- 2 apples, cored
- 1/4 cup chopped walnuts
- 1/2 teaspoon ground cinnamon
- Honey or maple syrup to taste (optional)
- Pinch of nutmeg (optional)

Instructions:

- Preheat oven to 375°F (190°C). Toss chopped walnuts with cinnamon and honey or maple syrup (if using).
- Fill the cored apples with the walnut mixture, sprinkle with nutmeg (if using).
- Place apples in a baking dish and bake for 20-25 minutes, or until tender and fragrant.

10. Coconut Chia Pudding with Mango and Pineapple

Ingredients:

- 1/4 cup chia seeds
- 1 cup unsweetened coconut milk
- 1/4 cup chopped mango

- 1/4 cup chopped pineapple
- 1/2 teaspoon vanilla extract
- Pinch of ground ginger (optional)
- Coconut flakes for garnish

Instructions:

- In a jar or container, whisk together chia seeds, coconut milk, vanilla extract, and ginger (if using).
- Stir in chopped mango and pineapple. Cover and refrigerate overnight.
- In the morning, the chia seeds will have absorbed the coconut milk and formed a pudding-like consistency.
- Garnish with additional mango, pineapple, and coconut flakes for a tropical and gut-friendly breakfast delight.
- Enjoy a naturally sweet and fiber-rich breakfast treat that's kind to your gut.

With these additions, you now have a complete Chapter 5 with 10 delicious and gut-friendly breakfast recipes! Remember, you can always adjust these recipes to your own preferences and dietary needs. Bon appetit, and happy gut-friendly mornings.

Chapter 5

Lunch Recipes

Lunchtime: that elusive hour when hunger meets mid-afternoon madness. However, the search for a nice and healthy lunch would be like passing many land mines through the path of a culinary minefield for people with IBD. Worry not, fellow adventurers! Chapter six is your sanctuary. Here you will find rich, delightful dishes that will be kind to your mind and body. Thus, put an appetite on, pin the apron on, and follow me in discovering mouth-watering lunches!

1. Rainbow Veggie Wraps with Hummus and Sprouts:

Ingredients:

- 2 whole wheat tortillas
- 1/4 cup hummus
- 1/2 cup mixed greens
- 1/4 cup shredded carrots
- 1/4 cup sliced cucumber
- 1/4 cup chopped red bell pepper
- 1/4 cup alfalfa sprouts

Instructions:

- Spread hummus evenly on each tortilla.
- Layer on the mixed greens, carrots, cucumber, and bell pepper.
- Top with a generous sprinkle of sprouts.
- Roll up tight and enjoy a colorful, crunchy lunch that's kind to your gut.

2. Salmon Salad with Quinoa and Lemon Dill Dressing:

Ingredients:

- 1 cup cooked quinoa
- 4 ounces baked or grilled salmon, flaked
- 1/2 cup chopped spinach
- 1/4 cup cherry tomatoes, halved
- 1/4 cup chopped red onion (optional) For the Dressing:
- 2 tablespoons olive oil
- 1 tablespoon lemon juice
- 1 teaspoon dill weed
- Salt and pepper to taste

Instructions:

- In a large bowl, combine quinoa, salmon, spinach, tomatoes, and red onion (if using).
- Whisk together olive oil, lemon juice, dill, salt, and pepper for the dressing.
- Drizzle the dressing over the salad and toss to combine.
- Enjoy a protein-packed and flavorful lunch that's gentle on your gut.

3. Curried Chickpea Salad Sandwiches on Whole Wheat Bread:

Ingredients:

- 1 can (15 oz) chickpeas, drained and rinsed
- 1/4 cup chopped red onion
- 1/4 cup chopped celery
- 2 tablespoons curry powder
- 1 tablespoon mayonnaise
- 1 tablespoon lemon juice
- Salt and pepper to taste

Instructions:

- Mash chickpeas with a fork until slightly chunky.
- Stir in red onion, celery, curry powder, mayonnaise, lemon juice, salt, and pepper.
- Spread on whole wheat bread and enjoy a satisfying and flavorful sandwich that's kind to your gut.

4. Lentil Soup with Whole Wheat Bread and Herbs:

Ingredients:

- 1 tablespoon olive oil
- 1 onion, chopped
- 2 cloves garlic, minced
- 1 cup green lentils, rinsed
- 4 cups vegetable broth
- 1 (14.5 oz) can diced tomatoes, undrained
- 1 teaspoon dried thyme
- 1/2 teaspoon dried oregano
- Salt and pepper to taste

Instructions:

- Heat olive oil in a large pot over medium heat. Add onion and cook until softened.
- Add garlic and cook for 30 seconds, stirring constantly.
- Stir in lentils, vegetable broth, diced tomatoes, thyme, oregano, salt, and pepper. Bring to a boil, then reduce heat and simmer for 20-30 minutes, or until lentils are tender.
- While the soup simmers, toast whole wheat bread for serving.

- Serve the lentil soup hot with toasted whole wheat bread and a sprinkle of fresh herbs (optional) for a simple and satisfying lunch that's kind to your gut.

5. Tuna Salad with Greek Yogurt and Avocado:

Ingredients:

- 2 cans (5 oz each) tuna, drained
- 1/4 cup plain Greek yogurt
- 1/4 cup chopped celery
- 1/4 cup chopped red onion
- 1 tablespoon lemon juice
- 1/2 avocado, mashed
- Salt and pepper to taste

Instructions:

- In a large bowl, combine tuna, Greek yogurt, celery, red onion, lemon juice, and mashed avocado.
- Season with salt and pepper to taste.
- Enjoy this protein-packed and creamy salad on whole wheat bread, lettuce wraps, or crackers for a satisfying and gut-friendly lunch.

6. Chicken Caesar Salad with Quinoa and Light Dressing:

Ingredients:

- 1 cup cooked quinoa
- 4 ounces grilled chicken, sliced
- 2 cups romaine lettuce, chopped
- 1/2 cup cherry tomatoes, halved
- 1/4 cup shaved Parmesan cheese For the Dressing
- 2 tablespoons olive oil
- 1 tablespoon lemon juice
- 1 teaspoon Dijon mustard
- 1/2 teaspoon garlic powder
- Salt and pepper to taste

Instructions:

- In a large bowl, combine quinoa, chicken, romaine lettuce, and cherry tomatoes.
- Whisk together olive oil, lemon juice, Dijon mustard, garlic powder, salt, and pepper for the dressing.
- Drizzle the dressing over the salad and toss to combine.
- Top with shaved Parmesan cheese and enjoy a light and flavorful salad that's kind to your gut.

7. Roasted Veggie Power Bowl with Quinoa and Tahini Dressing:

Ingredients:

- 1 cup cooked quinoa
- 1/2 cup roasted Brussels sprouts
- 1/2 cup roasted sweet potatoes, diced
- 1/4 cup roasted cauliflower florets
- 1/4 cup chopped red onion
- 1/4 cup chopped fresh parsley
- 2 tablespoons tahini
- 2 tablespoons lemon juice
- 1 tablespoon water
- 1 teaspoon olive oil
- Salt and pepper to taste

Instructions:

- Preheat oven to 400°F (200°C). Toss Brussels sprouts, sweet potatoes, and cauliflower with olive oil, salt, and pepper. Spread on a baking sheet and roast for 20-25 minutes, or until tender.

- In a bowl, combine cooked quinoa, roasted vegetables, red onion, and parsley.
- Whisk together tahini, lemon juice, water, olive oil, salt, and pepper for the dressing.
- Drizzle the dressing over the power bowl and enjoy a colorful and nourishing lunch that's kind to your gut.

8. Turkey and Veggie Lettuce Wraps with Cilantro Lime Ranch:

Ingredients:

- 4 large romaine lettuce leaves
- 4 ounces ground turkey, cooked
- 1/2 cup chopped bell peppers
- 1/2 cup shredded carrots
- 1/4 cup chopped red onion
- 1/4 cup chopped fresh cilantro

For the Cilantro Lime Ranch:

- 1/4 cup plain Greek yogurt
- 1/4 cup buttermilk
- 1 tablespoon lime juice
- 1 teaspoon chopped fresh cilantro
- Salt and pepper to taste

Instructions:

- Combine cooked ground turkey, bell peppers, carrots, red onion, and cilantro in a bowl.
- Whisk together yogurt, buttermilk, lime juice, cilantro, salt, and pepper for the dressing.
- Fill each romaine lettuce leaf with the turkey and veggie mixture. Drizzle with cilantro lime ranch dressing and enjoy a fresh and flavorful lunch that's kind to your gut.

9. Creamy Pumpkin Soup with Whole Wheat Bread Croutons:

Ingredients:

- 1 tablespoon olive oil
- 1 onion, chopped
- 2 cloves garlic, minced
- 4 cups vegetable broth
- 2 cups diced pumpkin
- 1/2 cup heavy cream (or substitute with coconut milk for a dairy-free option)
- 1 teaspoon dried sage
- Salt and pepper to taste

For the Croutons:

- 2 slices whole wheat bread, cubed
- 1 tablespoon olive oil
- Garlic powder and dried herbs (optional)

Instructions:

- Heat olive oil in a large pot over medium heat. Add onion and cook until softened.
- Add garlic and cook for 30 seconds, stirring constantly.
- Stir in vegetable broth, pumpkin, sage, salt, and pepper. Bring to a boil, then reduce heat and simmer for 20-25 minutes, or until pumpkin is tender.
- Remove from heat and puree with an immersion blender or in batches in a blender until smooth and creamy.
- Stir in heavy cream or coconut milk and warm through.
- While the soup simmers, prepare the croutons. Preheat oven to 375°F (190°C). Toss bread cubes with olive oil and season with garlic powder and dried herbs, if desired. Spread on a baking sheet and bake for 10-15 minutes, or until golden brown and crispy.
- Serve the creamy pumpkin soup hot with a sprinkle of whole wheat bread croutons for a comforting and gut-friendly lunch.

10. Mediterranean Chicken Skewers with Tzatziki Sauce:

Ingredients:

- 1 pound boneless, skinless chicken breast, cut into cubes
- 1/2 cup cherry tomatoes
- 1/2 cup red onion, cubed
- 1/4 cup crumbled feta cheese
- 1 tablespoon olive oil
- 1 teaspoon dried oregano
- 1/2 teaspoon garlic powder
- Salt and pepper to taste

For the Tzatziki Sauce:

- 1/2 cup plain Greek yogurt
- 1/4 cup chopped cucumber, drained
- 1 tablespoon lemon juice
- 1 teaspoon chopped fresh dill
- Salt and pepper to taste

Instructions:

- Preheat grill or grill pan to medium heat.
- Thread chicken, tomatoes, and red onion onto skewers.
- In a small bowl, whisk together olive oil, oregano, garlic powder, salt, and pepper. Brush onto the skewers.

- Grill skewers for 5-7 minutes per side, or until chicken is cooked through.

- While the skewers cook, prepare the tzatziki sauce by combining yogurt, cucumber, lemon juice, dill, salt, and pepper in a bowl.

- Serve chicken skewers with tzatziki sauce and enjoy a flavorful and gut-friendly lunch with a Mediterranean twist.

With these 10 delicious and gut-friendly lunch options, Chapter 5 is complete! Feel free to mix and match ingredients, explore new flavors, and discover your own culinary oasis. Remember, well-being starts from within, and a delicious and gut-friendly lunch is a step in the right direction. Bon appetit!

CHAPTER 6

Dinner Recipes

Gone are boring, monotonic meals that don't fulfill your taste and your belly. This is chapter seven that takes us through dinner as we embark on the journey of making our gut happy one bit at a time. It is about vibrant flavors, satisfying textures as well as friendly ingredients to the microbiota while at the same time offering zero moments of deprivation in the kitchen. Therefore, get hold of your apron and your cooking instincts, and be prepared to experience the wonders of a meal that not only fills one's stomach but also lifts one's spirit.

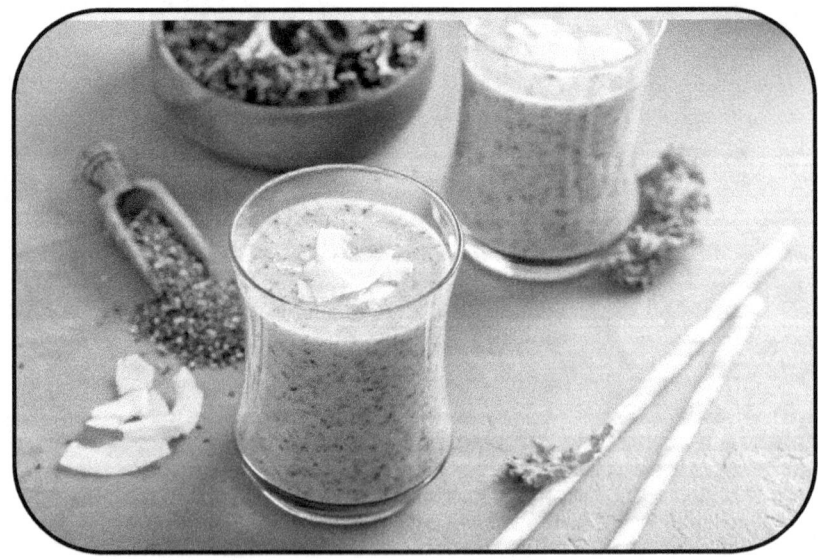

1. Salmon with Lemon-Ginger Glaze and Roasted Broccoli:

Ingredients:

- 1 salmon fillet (about 6 oz)
- 1 tablespoon olive oil
- 1/4 cup fresh lemon juice
- 1 tablespoon grated ginger
- 1/2 teaspoon honey
- Salt and pepper to taste
- 1 head broccoli, cut into florets

Instructions:

- Preheat oven to 400°F (200°C). Toss broccoli with olive oil, salt, and pepper. Spread on a baking sheet and roast for 15-20 minutes, or until tender-crisp.
- In a small bowl, whisk together lemon juice, ginger, honey, salt, and pepper.
- Heat olive oil in a skillet over medium heat. Sear salmon for 3-4 minutes per side, then brush with the lemon-ginger glaze.
- Continue cooking for 2-3 minutes, or until salmon is cooked through.

- Serve salmon with roasted broccoli and enjoy a gut-friendly and flavorful dinner.

2. One-Pan Turmeric Chicken with Sweet Potato and Peppers:

Ingredients:

- 4 boneless, skinless chicken thighs
- 1 tablespoon olive oil
- 1 teaspoon turmeric powder
- 1/2 teaspoon cumin powder
- 1/4 teaspoon paprika
- Salt and pepper to taste
- 1 medium sweet potato, diced
- 1 bell pepper, sliced
- 1/2 cup chicken broth

Instructions:

- Preheat oven to 425°F (220°C). Toss chicken with olive oil, turmeric, cumin, paprika, salt, and pepper.
- Arrange chicken, sweet potato, and bell pepper in a single layer on a baking sheet.
- Pour chicken broth into the bottom of the pan.

- Bake for 25-30 minutes, or until chicken is cooked through and vegetables are tender.
- Enjoy a warm and comforting one-pan meal that's kind to your gut!

3. Creamy Coconut Curry with Lentils and Spinach:

Ingredients:

- 1 tablespoon olive oil
- 1 medium onion, chopped
- 2 cloves garlic, minced
- 1 tablespoon curry powder
- 1 teaspoon ground ginger
- 1 can (14.5 oz) coconut milk
- 1 cup vegetable broth
- 1 cup green lentils, rinsed
- 4 cups chopped spinach
- Salt and pepper to taste

Instructions:

- Heat olive oil in a large pot over medium heat. Add onion and cook until softened.

- Add garlic, curry powder, and ginger, and cook for 1 minute, stirring constantly.
- Stir in coconut milk, vegetable broth, and lentils. Bring to a boil, then reduce heat and simmer for 20 minutes, or until lentils are tender.
- Stir in spinach and cook for 1-2 minutes, or until wilted. Season with salt and pepper to taste.
- Serve this flavorful and gut-friendly curry over brown rice or quinoa.

4. Vegetarian Chili with Brown Rice and Avocado:

Ingredients:

- 1 tablespoon olive oil
- 1 onion, chopped
- 2 cloves garlic, minced
- 1 (15 oz) can diced tomatoes
- 1 (15 oz) can black beans, rinsed and drained
- 1 (15 oz) can kidney beans, rinsed and drained
- 1 cup vegetable broth
- 1 teaspoon chili powder
- 1/2 teaspoon cumin powder
- 1/4 teaspoon smoked paprika

- Salt and pepper to taste
- 1 cup cooked brown rice
- 1 avocado, sliced

Instructions:

- Heat olive oil in a large pot over medium heat. Add onion and cook until softened.
- Add garlic and cook for 30 seconds, stirring constantly.
- Stir in diced tomatoes, black beans, kidney beans, vegetable broth, chili powder, cumin, paprika, salt, and pepper.
- Bring to a boil, then reduce heat and simmer for 20 minutes.
- Serve warm chili over cooked brown rice and top with sliced avocado for a delicious and gut-friendly meal.

5. Shrimp Scampi with Zucchini Noodles and Cherry Tomatoes:

Ingredients:

- 1 tablespoon olive oil
- 2 cloves garlic, minced
- 1/2 teaspoon red pepper flakes (optional)
- 1/4 cup white wine or chicken broth
- 1 pound large shrimp, peeled and deveined
- 1/2 cup cherry tomatoes, halved
- 1/4 cup chopped fresh parsley
- Salt and pepper to taste
- 2-3 zucchini, spiralized into noodles

Instructions:

- Heat olive oil in a large skillet over medium heat. Add garlic and red pepper flakes (if using) and cook for 30 seconds.
- Stir in white wine or chicken broth and bring to a simmer.
- Add shrimp and cook for 2-3 minutes per side, or until pink and opaque.
- Stir in cherry tomatoes and parsley and cook for 1 minute, or until tomatoes soften slightly. Season with salt and pepper to taste.

- Serve shrimp scampi over zucchini noodles for a low-carb and gut-friendly twist on a classic dish.

6. Baked Cod with Lemon Dill Sauce and Asparagus:

Ingredients:

- 2 cod fillets (about 6 oz each)
- 1 tablespoon olive oil
- Salt and pepper to taste
- 1/4 cup lemon juice
- 1/4 cup chopped fresh dill
- 1 pound asparagus, trimmed

Instructions:

- Preheat oven to 400°F (200°C). Line a baking sheet with parchment paper.
- Season cod fillets with salt and pepper.
- In a small bowl, whisk together lemon juice and dill.
- Brush half of the lemon dill sauce on the cod fillets.
- Place asparagus on the baking sheet and drizzle with olive oil. Season with salt and pepper.
- Arrange cod fillets on top of asparagus. Brush with remaining lemon dill sauce.

- Bake for 15-20 minutes, or until cod is cooked through and asparagus is tender-crisp.
- Serve this light and flavorful dish with your favorite sides.

7. Moroccan Chicken Tagine with Quinoa:

Ingredients:

- 1 tablespoon olive oil
- 1 onion, chopped
- 2 cloves garlic, minced
- 1 teaspoon ground turmeric
- 1/2 teaspoon ground ginger
- 1/4 teaspoon cinnamon
- Pinch of saffron (optional)
- 1 (14.5 oz) can diced tomatoes, undrained
- 1 cup chicken broth
- 4 boneless, skinless chicken thighs
- 1 cup cooked quinoa

Instructions:

- Heat olive oil in a large Dutch oven or ovenproof pot over medium heat. Add onion and cook until softened.

- Add garlic, turmeric, ginger, cinnamon, and saffron (if using) and cook for 30 seconds, stirring constantly.
- Stir in diced tomatoes and chicken broth. Bring to a simmer.
- Add chicken thighs and nestle them in the sauce. Cover and cook for 20-25 minutes, or until chicken is cooked through.
- Serve chicken tagine over cooked quinoa for a protein-packed and gut-friendly meal.

8. Mediterranean Salmon with Roasted Vegetables and Quinoa:

Ingredients:

- 2 salmon fillets (around 6 oz each)
- 1 tablespoon olive oil
- 1 teaspoon dried oregano
- 1/2 teaspoon garlic powder
- Salt and pepper to taste
- 1 zucchini, chopped
- 1 red bell pepper, chopped
- 1/2 red onion, sliced
- 1 cup quinoa, rinsed
- 1 1/2 cups vegetable broth

- 1/4 cup chopped fresh parsley (optional)

Instructions:

- Preheat oven to 400°F (200°C). Line a baking sheet with parchment paper.
- In a small bowl, combine olive oil, oregano, garlic powder, salt, and pepper. Rub the mixture onto the salmon fillets.
- Toss zucchini, bell pepper, and red onion with a drizzle of olive oil and arrange on the baking sheet. Place the salmon fillets on top.
- Roast for 15-20 minutes, or until the salmon is cook

9 . One-Pot Creamy Chicken Curry with Sweet Potato and Broccoli:

Ingredients:

- 1 tablespoon olive oil
- 1 pound boneless, skinless chicken thighs, cut into bite-sized pieces
- 1 onion, chopped
- 2 cloves garlic, minced
- 1 tablespoon curry powder
- 1 teaspoon ground turmeric
- 1/2 teaspoon ground ginger
- 1 (14.5 oz) can diced tomatoes, undrained

- 1 cup coconut milk
- 1 cup chicken broth
- 1 medium sweet potato, peeled and diced
- 1 head broccoli, cut into florets
- 1 cup cooked brown

Instructions:

- Heat olive oil in a large Dutch oven or pot over medium heat. Add the chicken and cook until browned on all sides.
- Stir in the onion and cook until softened, about 5 minutes. Add the garlic, curry powder, turmeric, and ginger, and cook for another minute, stirring constantly.
- Add the diced tomatoes, coconut milk, chicken broth, and sweet potato. Bring to a boil, then reduce heat

10. Salmon Burgers with Greek Yogurt Dill Sauce and Spiced Sweet Potato Fries:

Ingredients:

For the Burgers:

- 1 pound salmon fillets, skinless and chopped
- 1/4 cup breadcrumbs

- 1/4 cup chopped red onion
- 1 tablespoon chopped fresh dill
- 1/2 teaspoon lemon zest
- Salt and pepper to taste

For the Greek Yogurt Dill Sauce:

- 1/2 cup plain Greek yogurt
- 1 tablespoon chopped fresh dill
- 1 teaspoon lemon juice
- Salt and pepper to taste

For the Spiced Sweet Potato Fries:

- 2 medium sweet potatoes, peeled and cut into fries
- 1 tablespoon olive oil
- 1 teaspoon paprika
- 1/2 teaspoon cumin
- 1/4 teaspoon garlic powder
- Salt and pepper to taste

Instructions:

For the Burgers:

- Preheat oven to 400°F (200°C). Line a baking sheet with parchment paper.

- In a large bowl, combine salmon, breadcrumbs, red onion, dill, lemon zest, salt, and pepper. Mix well to form patties.
- Place salmon patties on the prepared baking sheet and bake for 15-20 minutes, or until cooked through.

Enjoy these delicious and gut-friendly dinner options! Remember, you can always adjust the ingredients and spices to your own preferences. Bon appetit!

CHAPTER 7

Dessert Recipes.

Need that sugary snack but not sure if it will affect your gut? Fear not, fellow adventurer! Gut-friendly goodness flows with flavor in chapter nine of this dessert desert. Bye-bye to bellyaches! Our sweet treats tango across your taste buds and coax your intestines with gentle words. Therefore, get your spoon out, be as greedy as possible, and lets venture into a realm full of delectable desserts which make both soul and body nutritious!

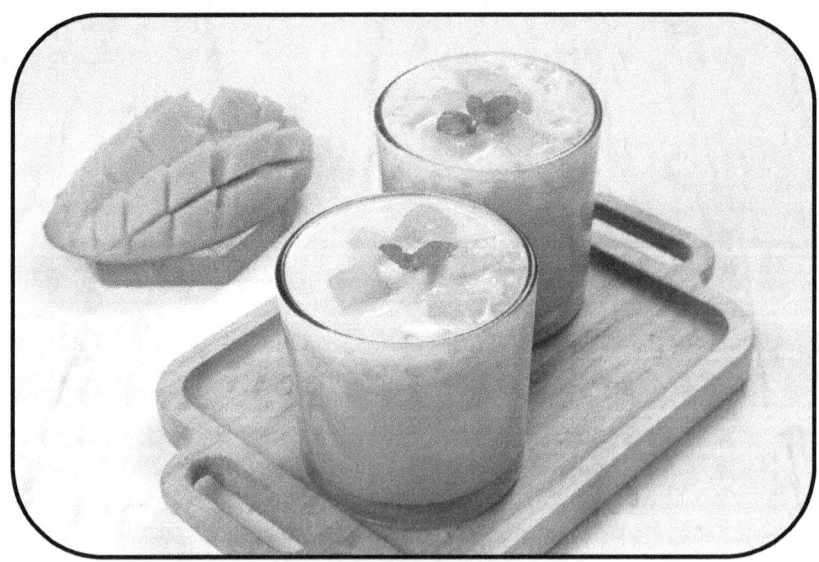

1. Creamy Chia Seed Pudding with Mango and Coconut

Ingredients:

- 1/4 cup chia seeds
- 1 cup unsweetened almond milk (or coconut milk for a dairy-free option)
- 1/2 ripe mango, diced
- 1/4 teaspoon vanilla extract
- 1 tablespoon shredded coconut (optional)

Instructions:

- Combine chia seeds, almond milk, and vanilla extract in a bowl or jar. Stir well and refrigerate overnight.
- In the morning, top your chia seed pudding with diced mango and sprinkle with shredded coconut (optional) for a creamy, tropical treat that's kind to your gut.

2. Baked Apples with Cinnamon and Walnuts

Ingredients:

- 2 apples, cored
- 1 tablespoon honey
- 1/2 teaspoon cinnamon
- 1/4 cup chopped walnuts

Instructions:

- Preheat oven to 375°F (190°C). Fill the apples with honey and cinnamon.
- Top with chopped walnuts and bake for 20-25 minutes, or until apples are tender and bubbly.
- Enjoy this warm and comforting dessert that's naturally sweet and gentle on your gut.

3. Frozen Yogurt Bites with Berries and Granola:

Ingredients:

- 1 cup plain Greek yogurt
- 1/4 cup mixed berries
- 1/4 cup granola

Instructions:

- Line a muffin tin with paper liners. Spoon Greek yogurt into each liner.
- Top with berries and sprinkle with granola. Freeze for 2-3 hours, or until solid.
- Enjoy these refreshing and portable frozen yogurt bites as a guilt-free sweet treat that's kind to your gut.

4. Dark Chocolate Bark with Almonds and Cranberries:

Ingredients:

- 1/2 cup dark chocolate chips
- 1/4 cup chopped almonds
- 01/4 cup dried cranberries

Instructions:

- Line a baking sheet with parchment paper. Melt dark chocolate in a microwave or double boiler.
- Pour melted chocolate onto the baking sheet and sprinkle with almonds and cranberries.
- Freeze for 15-20 minutes, then break into pieces for a satisfying and gut-friendly dessert with a rich, dark chocolate decadence.

5. Fruit Salad with Honey Lime Dressing:

Ingredients:

- Your favorite mix of fruits (berries, melon, mango, etc.)
- 1 tablespoon honey
- 1 tablespoon lime juice
- Mint leaves for garnish

Instructions:

- Toss your chosen fruits in a bowl.
- Whisk together honey and lime juice for a simple dressing.
- Drizzle the dressing over the fruit salad and garnish with mint leaves for a refreshing and light dessert that's kind to your gut.

6. Baked Pears with Ricotta and Honey:

Ingredients:

- 2 ripe pears, halved and cored
- 1/4 cup ricotta cheese
- 1/4 teaspoon cinnamon
- 1 tablespoon honey
- Chopped walnuts or pecans (optional)

Instructions:

- Preheat oven to 375°F (190°C). Fill pear halves with ricotta cheese and sprinkle with cinnamon.
- Drizzle with honey and bake for 20-25 minutes, or until pears are tender and bubbly.
- Top with chopped walnuts or pecans for a warm and comforting dessert that's rich in protein and gentle on your gut.

7. Creamy Coconut Rice Pudding with Mango:

Ingredients:

- 1/2 cup cooked brown rice
- 1 cup coconut milk
- 1/4 cup chopped mango
- 1 tablespoon maple syrup
- Pinch of cardamom powder
- Fresh mint leaves for garnish (optional)

Instructions:

- In a saucepan, combine cooked rice, coconut milk, mango, maple syrup, and cardamom powder. Bring to a simmer and cook for 5 minutes, stirring occasionally.

- Remove from heat and let cool slightly. Garnish with fresh mint leaves for a tropical treat that's creamy, fragrant, and kind to your gut.

8. No-Bake Dark Chocolate Mousse with Berries:

Ingredients:

- 1 cup full-fat canned coconut milk, chilled overnight
- 1/4 cup melted dark chocolate
- 1 tablespoon maple syrup
- Pinch of sea salt
- Fresh berries for topping

Instructions:

- Scoop out the solidified coconut cream from the can and whip it until light and fluffy.
- Gently fold in melted chocolate, maple syrup, and sea salt.
- Spoon the mousse into individual glasses and top with fresh berries for a decadent and gut-friendly dessert that requires no baking.

9. Spiced Roasted Sweet Potato with Coconut Yogurt and Berries:

Ingredients:

- 1 small sweet potato, peeled and diced
- 1 tablespoon olive oil
- 1/2 teaspoon cinnamon
- Pinch of nutmeg
- 1/4 cup plain Greek yogurt
- 1 tablespoon shredded coconut
- Fresh berries for topping

Instructions:

- Preheat oven to 400°F (200°C). Toss sweet potato cubes with olive oil, cinnamon, and nutmeg.
- Spread on a baking sheet and roast for 20-25 minutes, or until tender and golden brown.
- Top with a dollop of Greek yogurt, sprinkle with shredded coconut, and finish with fresh berries for a satisfying and gut-friendly dessert that's naturally sweet and packed with nutrients.

10. Fruit Smoothie with Spinach and Yogurt

Ingredients:

- 1 cup frozen mixed berries
- 1/2 cup spinach
- 1/2 cup plain Greek yogurt
- 1/4 cup unsweetened almond milk (optional)
- 1 teaspoon honey (optional)

Instructions:

- Blend together all ingredients until smooth and creamy. Add more almond milk or honey for desired consistency and sweetness.

- Enjoy this refreshing and energizing smoothie as a perfect post-dinner dessert or a guilt-free snack that's packed with vitamins and gentle on your gut.

With this final set of recipes, Chapter 7 is complete. Remember, there are endless possibilities for crafting delicious and gut-friendly desserts. So, go forth and experiment, explore new flavors, and discover what satisfies your sweet tooth while nourishing your body and soul. Bon appetit, and happy indulging!

Chapter 8

Meal Planning and Preparation

You can't win over your IBD while saying goodbye to appetizing and filling foods, you know. Surprisingly, if properly planned for, your kitchen could become a sanctuary of nourishment for both body and soul; packed with healthy nutrients that are beneficial to the digestive system. Okay then, put on your apron, sharpen your knives, and get started with the seven-day culinary voyage!

PLANNING WITH PURPOSE

Know your triggers: Evaluate what food items are likely to trigger a flare in your IBD. Try including them in your menu but do not base it on their dietary fiber value. Instead, prefer gut-friendly staples such as lean proteins, fruits, vegetables, and whole grains.

- **Embrace variety:** Never stick into your comfort zone! Try out with various cuisines and textures to ensure your mouth stays entertained, while your digestive system is content.
- **Time is your friend:** Batch cook whenever possible. For example, if you're roasting a whole chicken or making a large pot of soup over the weekends you'll see that the

results pay off during the week as it will save you both time and energy.

- **Leftovers are your allies:** Prepare simple meals, which can also be changed into flavorful re-heated snacks for your lunch/next fast meal.
- **Don't forget snacks:** Store healthy snacks such as nuts, fruit and yoghurt easily accessible so they can stave off unhealthy food temptation when hunger arises.

PREPARATION MADE EASY

Shop smart: And don't be too ambitious. Write them down, make your shopping lists!! Don't make any "on-the-gut" purchases.

- **Chop like a pro:** Spend about five minutes chopping the vegetables, seal them into airtight bags for easy storage.
- **Marinate your magic:** Overnight marination of meat, tofu or veggie makes them easier to digest while enhancing their taste and tenderness at the same time.
- **Befriend your freezer:** Cook extra food so that you can take some portions and freeze them for the next time when you don't have enough time.
- **Utilize technology:** Buy yourself a crock pot or Instant Pot to help with cooking and save time.

RESOURCES FOR IBD-FRIENDLY MEAL PLANS

The Crohn's & Colitis Foundation: Provides a whole lot of information and materials such as gut friendly recipes with guidelines and meal plans.

The National Digestive Diseases Information Clearinghouse: Reliable info and products about digestive disorders, including IBD dietary recommendations.

Apps like "Mealtime" and "Eat This Much": Provide customised meal scheduling suggestions with respect to dietary limitations/preferences as well as items suited for IBD.

Cookbooks like "The Complete Idiot's Guide to Living Well with Crohn's Disease" and "The IBD Cookbook": Offer tasty recipes that have easy instructions which can be digested by people suffering from IBD.

To recap, meal planning and prepping is not about strict rules or confines. Its about trying out the best system or method that fits in your time schedule and your gut feeling also. Have fun! Use your imagination. Try different flavors. Before long will have you serving healthy gut-pleasers that not only taste fantastic but do wonders for your insides. Bon appetit, and happy cooking!

Your cooking journey starts with this chapter. Keep posted on more advises, ideas, recipes and other useful material regarding cooking to care for your health inside-out!

How to Plan Meals for the Week:

Fear not, fellow IBD warriors! Meal planning doesn't have to be a daunting chore. With a little organization and these simple steps, you can create a weekly menu that's both delicious and kind to your gut:

1. Gather inspiration:

Browse cookbooks and online resources: Explore dedicated IBD-friendly recipe websites, cookbooks, and social media groups for fresh ideas.

Consider your cravings: Think about meals you enjoy and translate them into gut-friendly versions.

Utilize leftover magic: Plan meals that can easily be transformed into leftovers for the next day or another quick lunch.

Seasonal bounty: Prioritize fresh, seasonal ingredients for optimal flavor and nutrition.

2. Take inventory:

Pantry audit: Check your pantry and fridge for staples like whole grains, protein sources, fruits, and vegetables.

Identify limitations: Note any ingredients that tend to trigger your IBD and make sure to avoid them.

Make a shopping list: Stick to your list to avoid impulse purchases that might not be gut-friendly.

3. Time-saving tricks:

Batch cooking: Dedicate a weekend morning to prepping ingredients or cooking large batches of soup, grains, or proteins for the week.

Chop and store: Chop vegetables and fruits in advance and store them in airtight containers for quick access.

Embrace the freezer: Portion out and freeze cooked meals for instant satisfaction on busy nights.

Delegate tasks: If possible, involve family or friends in the planning and preparation process.

4. Build your weekly menu:

Balance is key: Aim for a variety of meals including protein, complex carbohydrates, healthy fats, and plenty of fruits and vegetables.

Theme nights: Spice things up with designated theme nights like **"Meatless Mondays" or "Taco Tuesdays."**

Don't forget snacks: Plan healthy snacks like nuts, yogurt, or fruit slices to avoid unhealthy temptations when hunger strikes.

Flexibility matters: Leave room for adjustments based on your energy levels and schedule throughout the week.

5. Tools for success:

- **Meal planning apps:** Utilize apps like "Mealime" or "Eat This Much" to create personalized menus based on your dietary needs and preferences.
- **Printable templates:** Download or create your own weekly meal planner templates to keep track of your menu and grocery list.
- **Get creative:** Don't be afraid to experiment with new ingredients and flavors! The more you enjoy the process, the more likely you are to stick to your plan.

Remember, meal planning is a journey, not a destination. Be patient, experiment, and most importantly, have fun! With these tips and a little practice, you'll be whipping up gut-friendly masterpieces that nourish your body and soul in no time.

Tips for making meal preparation easier

You have a weekly menu with you and it's time to attack the kitchen. However, my fellow IBD warriors, prepping meals is not a full-scale endurance race! Here are some tips to streamline the process and make it a breeze:

1. Embrace the power of multitasking:

- **Chop while it simmers:** In addition, you can take advantage of the bubbling stage and cut veggies for different snacks and main courses.

- **Multigrain madness:** Simultaneously cook several types of grain for various dishes across this week. Versatile you have brown rice, versatile you have quinoa.

- **Double duty dishes:** Cook whole chicken for dinner and use it as an ingredient in salad, sandwich or vegetable stir-fry.

2. Utilize the power of technology:

- **Slow cooker magic:** Add your ingredients in the morning and have a prepared meal to eat upon getting home.

- **Instant Pot power**. You will save time in your kitchen with this multi-cooker that can pressure cook, steam, and sauté.

- **Food processors and blenders:** They are very convenient for chopping vegetables, pureeing of soups, making healthy nut butter, among other numerous reasons.

3. Organize your workspace:

- **Declutter your counters:** Don't clutter the space to prevent frustration and improve cooking experience.
- **Sharpen your tools:** Dull knives make everything harder. Always ensure you keep your knives in tip top condition for easy, safe chopping.
- **Containerize chaos:** Pre-portioned items should be stored in leak proof containers which will ensure everything is still fresh and organized

4. Prep like a pro:

- **Wash and chop in bulk:** Schedule a certain period of the entire week exclusively for washing, cutting, cleaning all varieties of fruits and vegetables.
- **Marinate your way to success:** To have better taste and for easy absorption of digested food in the body.
- **Portion control is key:** Separate cooked food into single portions that can be grabbed and eaten as takeaways or during a rushed supper.

5. Don't be afraid to delegate:

- **Involve the family:** Involve your family in the cooking and make it into an exciting and bonding activity.

- **Utilize leftovers:** Plan to cook meals that you can use as snacks and lunch for the following day, cutting down on your preparation time.

So remember, meals are all about making it work for you. Do not hesitate to mix things up and tailor these tips to suit you. In no time, you'll be a king or queen of your kitchen making bowel sensitive foods at your own ease.

CHAPTER 9

Living with IBD.

IBD is not an easy buddy, but it need not define who you are. Herein, this chapter becomes the map through which you will learn how to handle the IBD and attain overall healthiness even as you experience bliss. Just remember that you are not traveling alone to your destination.

Tips for Managing IBD Symptoms:

Listen to your body: Be aware of what makes you tick and change your diets, stressors, and exercise routines as appropriate.

Embrace gut-friendly foods: Choose whole grain food, lean proteins, fresh fruit and veggies, while reducing intake of processed food, sugar-drinks and fattening dishes.8pgfscope

Stay hydrated: Water is your best friend! Make sure you take at least 8 glasses of water in a day for better functioning of your body.

Stress management is key: Try out yoga, meditation, and taking a walk outside in order to healthily manage your stress levels.

Sleep for healing: Good sleep hygiene should be prioritized by making sure you have a regular sleeping pattern and calming bedtime routine.

Medications and treatments: It is advisable to strictly follow your physician's prescription and inquiries regarding the dosage and the expected outcome of medicines.

Connect with your community: In addition, surround yourself with a support group of friends and family members that can encourage you while sharing similar experiences.

Resources for IBD Support:

The Crohn's & Colitis Foundation: The premier entity in the provision of necessary literature, support systems and training sessions for those suffering from IBD.

- **National Digestive Diseases Information Clearinghouse:** It is a trustworthy and current government's website giving details about IBD as one of the digestion disorders.
- **Online communities and forums:** Use online forums and social media groups as platforms where you can find peers who share some of your experiences and give some kind of support like understanding or sharing advice.

Mental health resources: Taking care of IBD is not easy at all in terms of an emotional perspective. Do not forget that it is always possible to get professional help.

Wellness and fitness resources: Identify activities and exercise you love that encourage general health.

Living Life to the Fullest with IBD

- **Focus on what you can control:** Don't let IBD control you. Focus on the things you can influence, like your diet, stress levels, and attitude.

- **Embrace small victories:** Celebrate every step forward, no matter how small. Each positive change is a win on your journey.
- **Find your passion:** Pursue activities that bring you joy and purpose, whether it's through hobbies, creative pursuits, or meaningful connections.
- **Travel and explore:** Don't let IBD limit your travel dreams. Plan trips with your condition in mind and enjoy new experiences.
- **Advocate for yourself:** Be proactive in your healthcare by asking questions, researching options, and participating in clinical trials.

Remember, you are strong and resilient. You have the power to overcome challenges and live a fulfilling life with IBD. Never give up on yourself!

Together, let's rewrite the narrative of IBD and turn it into a story of resilience, strength, and living life to the fullest!

CONCLUSION

As you turn the last page, my dear reader, let us step away from the stove and relish the last vestiges of this culinary adventure. You've danced with spices that calm your stomach and excite your taste buds, vanquished monsters of meal planning, and explored mountains of bright cuisine. Keep in mind that you are about to go on a journey beyond boring with this cookbook.

Take a deep breath, enjoy the feast you've made, and grin. You've demonstrated that tasty and suitable for those with inflammatory bowel disease (IBD) can coexist. Your kitchen is now a sanctuary of digestive delight, and your body is dancing in blissful silence.

The journey, however, is far from over. Use this cookbook as a guide to limitless culinary adventures; it's a reliable friend in the kitchen. Never allow IBD extinguish your passion for cooking; instead, explore, innovate, and give your own unique spin to these recipes. Just keep in mind that every mouthful is sending a message to your taste buds that they are deserving of a celebration and to your tummy that it's okay to join in on the celebration.

Thus, fearless eater, go forward! Inform people, show them what you can make, and encourage them to take control of their kitchens and inflammatory bowel disease (IBD) by sharing your recipes.

Remember the tantalizing aromas and the joy in your gut the next time self-doubt creeps in, and you will be certain that you are in control of your own wonderful fate.

May your culinary adventures be filled with joy, laughter, and love from the inside out! Bon appétit!

Instead of a sigh, let the cookbook finish with one last flourish, accompanied by the sound of spoons clink and the chorus of satisfied bellies. The journey is only at its start!